Foot Health – Pamper Your Feet!

Take Care of Your Feet to Reduce

Diabetes-Related Foot Issues

RON KNESS

Brought to You

By **Diabetes Management** at

https://healthylifestylenewsletter.com/diabetes

Published by:

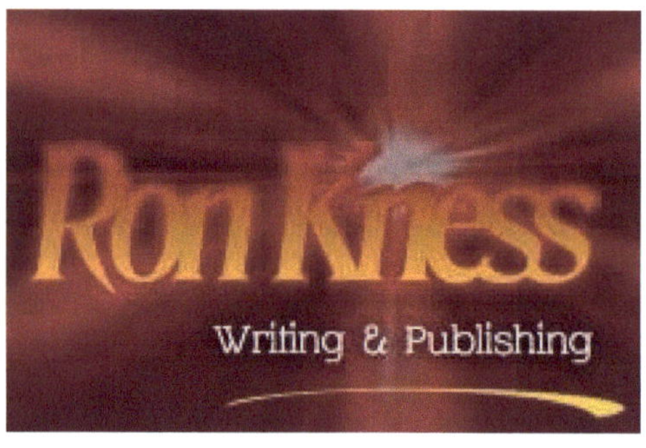

Gold Canyon, AZ

United States of America

ISBN-13: 978-1976137648

ISBN-10: 1976137640

Contents

Disclaimer

This publication is for informational purposes only and is not intended as medical advice. Medical advice should always be obtained from a qualified medical professional for any health conditions or symptoms associated with them.

Every possible effort has been made in preparing and researching this material. We make no warranties with respect to the accuracy, applicability of its contents or any omissions.

See your healthcare professional before starting any diet, health or exercise program!

Foot Health - Pamper Your Feet

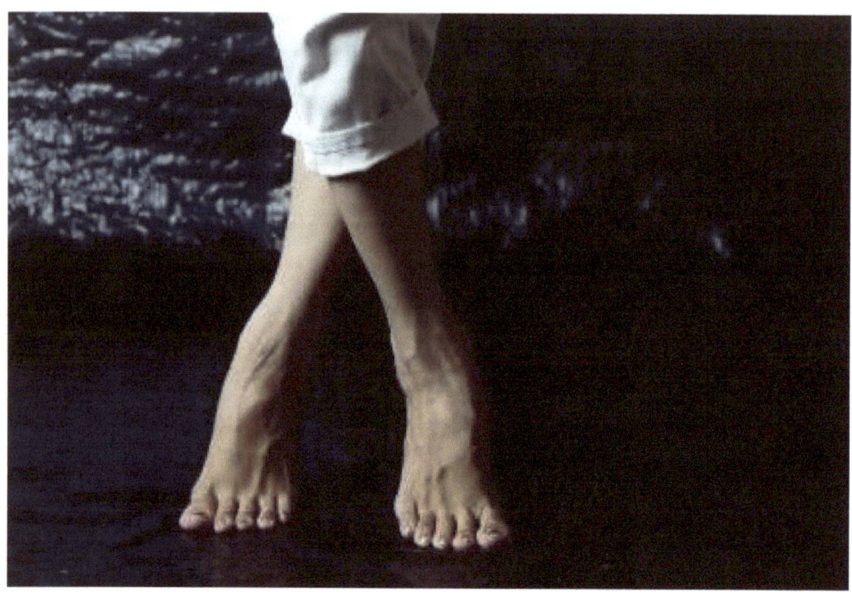

Having healthy feet, and keeping them as pain free as possible, is important to be physically active. It doesn't matter if you're trying to prevent problems or you already have problems, taking care of your feet is imperative. Especially if you want to be involved in fun physical activities like walking, jogging, dancing, and playing sports. Even if you just want to be able to walk for your entire life, foot health is essential.

Potential Foot Problems

Many foot problems can be avoided, but some are purely the luck of genetics. Let's go over the various types of foot problems that many people encounter over their lifetime.

- **Athlete's Foot** – Some people mistakenly think that they have dry skin when they really have Athlete's Foot. Athlete's Foot is caused by a fungus. Most fungi love dark, warm, moist places. Your feet, especially between your toes, is prime real-estate for it to take hold.

- **Hammertoes** – This can be prevented. It looks like all the toes are smashed together and bent permanently. This can be very painful. It's caused by wearing ill-fitting shoes throughout your lifetime. Make sure that your shoes fit right. Don't shove your feet into a shoe that doesn't fit properly or pointy-toed shoes, just to fit in with fashion.

- **Blisters** – Caused by ill-fitting and fashionable shoes. Blisters are soft pockets of skin filled with water, giving them a raised appearance. Blisters should be properly drained and bandaged. But prevention is the key. Wear only well-fitting shoes and if you sweat, change your socks often.

- **Bunions** – This is a crooked big toe joint that kind of sticks out forcing the big toe to turn in somewhat, but the joint sticks out uncomfortably often getting rubbed by even shoes that fit well. Often wearing narrow shoes is the cause of bunions. Surgery could be a possibility for relief.

- **Corns & Calluses** – Caused by repetitive rubbing of an area against something else, usually against a shoe. Corns are on the top of your feet and calluses appear on the bottom of your feet. You can prevent this by wearing shoes that fit. If they're really bad, and are painful, a doctor should remove them.

- **Plantar Fasciitis** – This condition happens when tissue connected to the ball part of the heel becomes inflamed. The best way to treat this is medically, but well-fitting shoes that have heel padding can help. It can be very painful.

- **Claw Toes** – This is caused by diabetes, arthritis, and other health problems along with wearing ill-fitting or inappropriate shoes. Nerve damage to feet, due to illness, is more likely the culprit, but it can happen to anyone. If you have this problem seek immediate medical care for your feet.

- **Gout** – This is a condition caused by a buildup of uric acid in the joints. While gout can affect any joint in your body it usually affects the big toe.

  If your big toe gets warm, red, swollen and is very painful, even if a sock or blanket is on the toe, it's probably gout. This requires medical intervention because the pain is so intense. Try adding tart cherry juice or pills and eat a low purine diet to lower your uric acid levels. However, medication is generally needed.

- **Ingrown Nails** – This is usually caused by cutting your nails wrong, an injury to the nail, or poorly fitting shoes. What happens is that the nail starts growing toward the skin on the edge of the nail which becomes red and inflamed. It can become very infected if not treated properly. Cut nails straight across, and not too short, to avoid causing ingrown nails.

- **Nail Fungus** – Nail fungus is the bane of many people's existence. It causes embarrassment, due to its ugly deformed appearance. It's near impossible to avoid it, too.

Don't walk around barefoot in public areas, showers, gyms, and hotel rooms. There are some treatments that show promise, like laser treatment and entire nail removal. Some prescription drugs work for some people, but the side effects may not be worth it.

Improve Foot Health

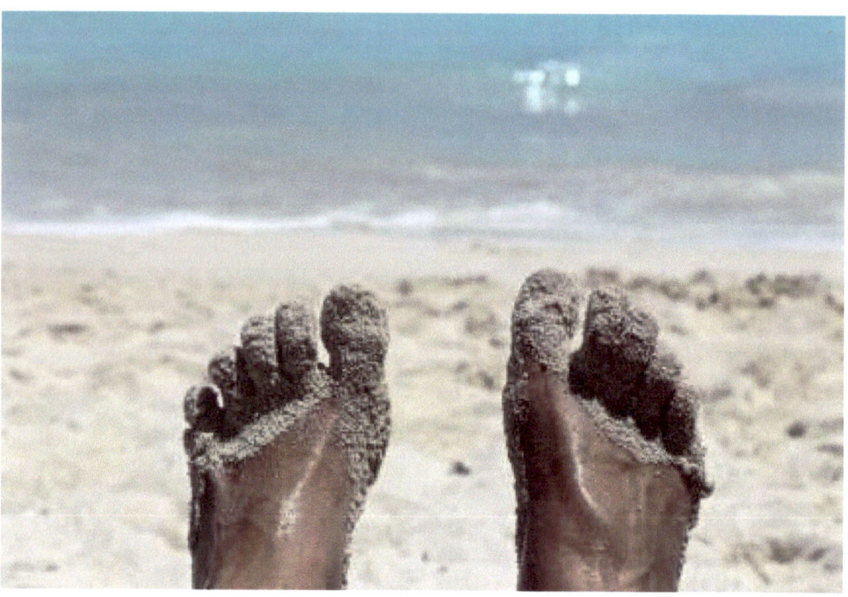

To keep your feet as healthy as possible, for as long as possible, let's learn everything we can that affects foot health and what you can do to improve it. After all, you need your feet 365 days a year, 24 hours a day, 7 days a week … for life. Proper foot care can mean the difference between a lifetime of happy feet or painful feet or in the case of diabetics – amputation of a foot or lower part of a leg.

Increase Blood Flow

One issue with feet is a lack of blood flow. The best way to ensure adequate blood flow to your feet is to exercise your feet. Walking is a good exercise for feet.

If you have a sedentary job you'll need to try to find ways to wiggle your feet and toes to keep the blood flowing. Spread your toes, and wiggle them often, to keep the blood flowing. If you cross your legs when sitting, switch often to allow the blood to flow freely. Get, or give yourself, regular foot massages.

Manage Your Weight

While every single problem a person has can't be traced back to weight when it comes to your feet, if you have swelling and painful feet and are overweight, you may see a huge improvement if you drop to a healthy weight. Remember all your weight is on your feet, and that is compounded with each step, depending on how fast you are moving.

Weight management starts with eating right. In fact, even if your feet currently hurt too much to walk on them, you can still lose weight which may help your painful feet. Eat a diet as close to nature as possible, avoiding processed food. Drink plenty of fresh, filtered water, and remember it really is about calories in and calories out, no matter what anyone else says.

Going Barefoot - Yes or No?

Like any advice, whether medical or non-medical, the case for going barefoot has its pros and its cons.

It's recommended that children be allowed to go barefoot as much as possible. It helps them develop through the stimuli experienced through their feet. It also helps them to be more aware of the environment they are in.

Feet need fresh air and the toes need to be allowed to spread out in a natural pattern. Placing the feet into shoes is actually unnatural, though shoes do offer more protection than going barefoot.

Yoga and martial arts are all practiced barefoot. These practices have been around for hundreds, if not thousands, of years.

If you have diabetes, or serious foot conditions, you may want to keep your shoes on. However, it's probably very beneficial to you if you can go barefoot around your home, and even in your own yard where you know it's clean of debris and there's no risk of stepping on glass, thorns or any other sharp objects.

In the medical community, you find many doctors who suggest going barefoot, while just as many others suggest you should never go barefoot. The decision may be up to you and what you feel most comfortable with.

If you enjoy having your feet free from shoes, especially in your own home, by all means do it. If you feel more comfortable keeping your shoes on, except for in bed, then do that.

Pamper Your Feet

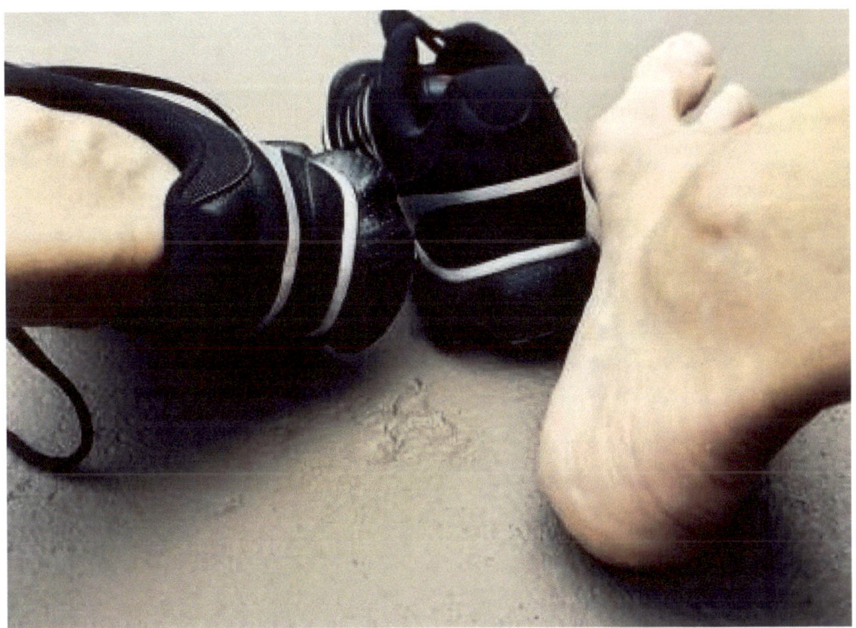

It's important that you practice proper daily foot care. That will ensure that you don't have any problems surfacing that need immediate care. This is more important as you get older, but if you develop the habit now you'll keep it for a lifetime.

- **Keep Them Clean** – Every day, wash your feet with warm soapy water. Dry thoroughly, then apply lotion that is made for feet. Choose a lotion that is natural, without a lot of perfumes and alcohol in it. That way your feet will get soft and not accidentally dried out.

- **Wear Clean Socks** – Socks should be clean, cotton, and preferably white most of the time. Sure, you can get into fashion occasionally, but understand that when you're walking or working out, white cotton socks that fit your feet snugly but not too tightly, are best.

- **Keep Them Dry** – If you work in a job where your feet sweat, bring a couple extra pairs of socks so that you can change your socks during the day. Nothing is worse than walking around in soggy socks. It can cause fungus, calluses, ulcers and more problems to walk around with wet soggy feet.

- **Wear Well Fitting Shoes** – If you're not sure what a well-fitting shoe is, go to an upscale shoe store to help size you properly. Buying shoes from discount stores can often be great on your wallet today, but in the long run, probably won't help your feet or your wallet when you have increased healthcare costs due to wearing ill-fitting, poorly made shoes.

- **Shoe Style** – Wearing foot protection (shoes) is imperative, especially outdoors. Wearing flip flops, flats without support, or other slippers – none of these are good for providing protection to your feet. Chiropractors see more back issues from people wearing flip-flops than they do from any other shoe. There are also record numbers of sprained ankles and broken ankles from wearing flip-flops.

- **Don't Sit Too Long** – It might seem counterintuitive but sitting can be very bad for your foot health. The reason is that you need blood flow to your feet and sitting can impede that depending on how you sit.

If you do have to sit a lot find ways to exercise your feet, move your legs, and go for walks during the day.

- **Check Your Feet Daily** – Every single day, when you wash your feet, check them out. Look between your toes, on the bottom of your feet, (use a mirror) checking for issues such as fungus, calluses, ulcers and other issues that could become bigger problems and deal with them right then.

- **Trim Toenails Correctly** – One problem with how people care for their feet today is how people trim their toenails. This is especially true if you tend to get pedicures by the "so-called" professionals. Some places trim nails wrong.

You are only supposed to trim nails straight across with a proper nail clipper, and then file the edge to avoid sharp areas. You're not supposed to cut into the corners of your toenails. This can cause a nasty ingrown toenail and infection.

Keeping your feet dry, in the right-sized shoes, and clean, is important for good foot care. When you pamper your feet, you're really pampering your entire body. When your feet feel good, you feel good.

Foot Care Warning Signs

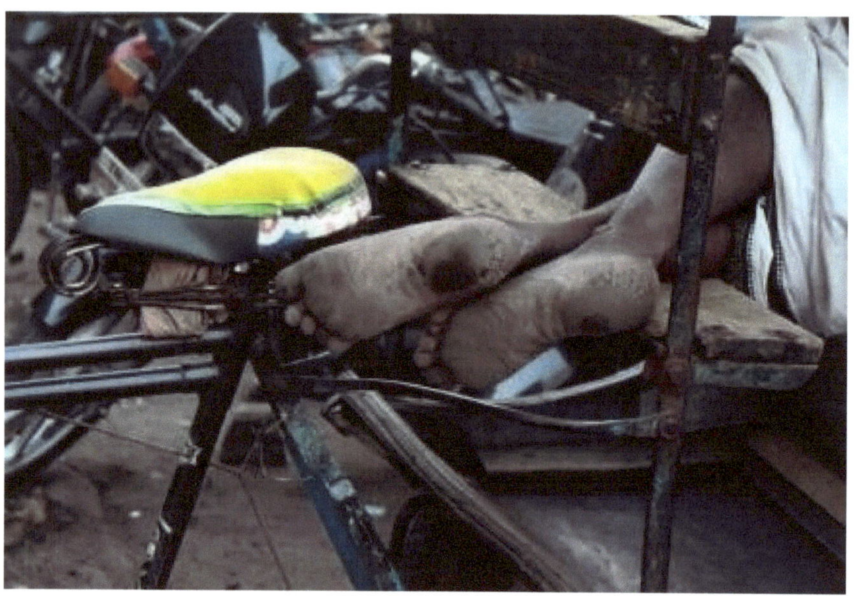

If you are paying attention to your feet daily, you will notice signs of problems that may need professional help. It cannot be stressed enough how important foot care is. Pampering your feet will keep your feet healthy your entire life. If you do have issues, these warning signs will signal that you should seek medical intervention sooner than if you ignore your feet and don't practice some type of daily care.

Lack of Sensation (or extra sensation) – If you ever notice any lack of sensation in your feet, whether it's pins and needles feeling, or worse like bees stinging you, you might have something called neuropathy.

This is not uncommon for people with diabetes or other issues and requires medical attention.

Ulcers – If you have ulcers on your feet which typically start in calluses left untreated and uncleaned, then you should seek immediate medical care to ensure that the ulcer is treated before you get an infection that can get into your bloodstream and cause serious health issues, amputation, and even death.

Ingrown Toenails – If you get ingrown toenails often, you should go see a foot doctor. They will teach you the proper way to cut your nails to help you avoid additional issues and they can also treat the current ingrown toenail to help you prevent serious infection.

Pain – Feet aren't really supposed to hurt all the time. If you're having issues standing or walking due to foot pain, regardless of location, it's imperative to seek the assistance of a podiatrist. They will analyze all your problems from how you walk, the shoes you wear, how you care for your feet and other health problems such as diabetes that can cause foot problems.

If you have any of these warning signs, seek immediate medical attention with your podiatrist or general practitioner who may send you a referral to a podiatrist. Thankfully, there are many things you can do at home to prevent having to go to the doctor too often.

Choosing the Right Shoes

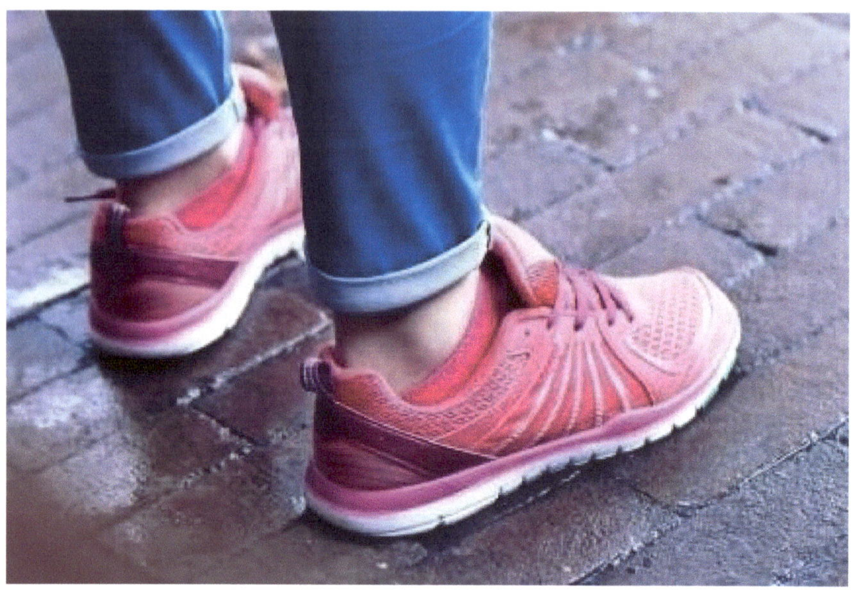

Shoes are so important. Picking the right size and shape for your foot and for the reason you're buying the shoes is important to good foot health. While it may seem fun to go with the fun fashions, doing so regularly can cause a lifetime of problems.

Even if those pointy high heels don't hurt today, they are damaging your feet now (and your back) and you'll suffer for it as you age. If you must wear a certain type of shoe, due to work, find a good orthopedic shoe store. You may be surprised that they do have good shoes that will fit with your dress code and save your feet, too.

Check the Size

Don't try to keep wearing the same size of shoe your entire life. Your feet keep growing and changing as you age. Get your feet measured by a professional toward the end of the day to get an accurate size since that's the time your feet are at their largest.

Go by how they feel rather than the number. That's just a starting point, since all shoes are made differently. Plus, if you have one foot larger than the other, get shoes to fit the largest foot.

Check the Shape

Most people should wear shoes that are shaped like their own feet for maximum comfort and fit. If you have pointy toes, you can wear shoes with pointy toes but if you have a square toe you'll need shoes shaped that way. You don't want to shove your foot into a shoe that forces your foot to form to the shape.

Check the Fit

When you're checking the fit the common rule of thumb, according to WebMD, is that you should have about ½ inch of space between your longest toe and the front of the toe box in the shoe when standing.

Plus, the ball of your foot should fit easily into the widest part of the shoe and the heel should not slip or ride up and down on your feet when you walk. Shoes don't stretch to fit and you don't need to "break-in" shoes, they should fit and feel comfortable from day one. If they're not fitting right or comfortable the day you buy them, they never will be.

Check the Material

The best material for shoes is leather, but there are new materials being created every day that will also work if you're opposed to leather. The important thing is that the material is soft and flexible and will mold to and match the shape of your foot with wear. The soles of the shoes shouldn't be slippery and should cushion your feet from the pressure of walking on hard surfaces. If possible, avoid high heels.

Ask Your Podiatrist

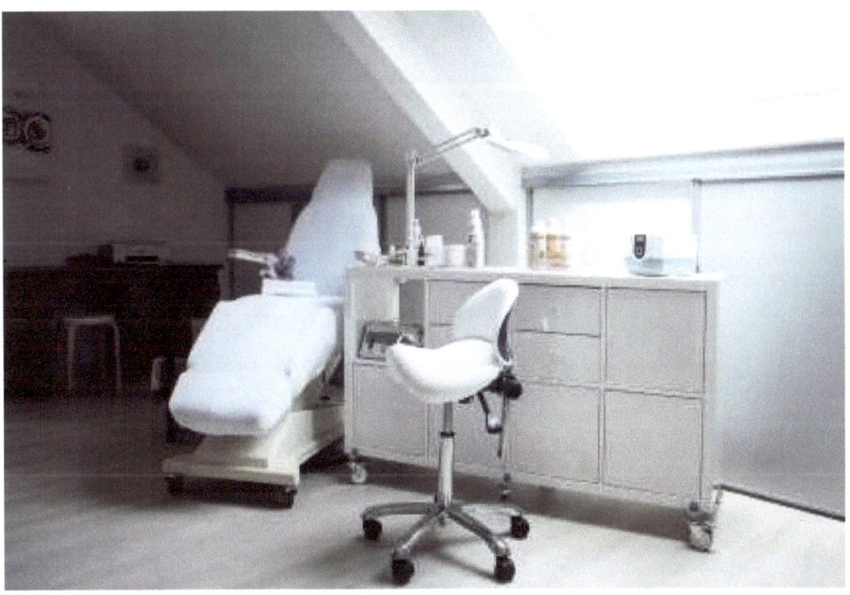

A doctor can give you a list of brands of shoes for you to try that are made correctly and help cut down on foot pain and problems. Shoes like Birkenstocks, Crocs, Rainbow, and others offer great options. The important part is that the shoe offers the right support for your arch and your heel, and that they feel good when you're walking and giving you protection between the ground and your foot.

If you think of your shoes as an investment, you will be able to buy shoes that last. If you wear shoes daily though, like for sports, you'll need to replace them every six months to a year. Look for sales, learn which brands work for you, and you'll be able to pick the right shoes for the best foot health.

When to See a Podiatrist

There are times when you may need to seek the assistance of a podiatrist. Most people tend to just tough it out and try to care for their feet themselves. Later we will talk about some non-medical treatments that can help but there are times when you should consider seeing a podiatrist to help you pamper your feet the best.

- **Persistent Pain** – Corns, heel spurs, and other issues can start to cause severe and persistent pain in your feet that get in the way of your daily life. Any pain, no matter the reason, should be checked by your doctor because there may be ways to treat it so you can get relief.

- **Changes in Your Nails** – If your nails change in color, it could be either fungus or it could even be cancer. It's best to get any strange changes in color diagnosed by a professional. People have died from skin cancer that started under their toenails.

- **Skin Changes on Your Feet** – When you check your feet daily, you'll be aware of any issues or changes. If you see yellowing of nails, changes in skin color and texture or other signs, seek medical attention. These can be signs of infections that need medicine you can't get over the counter.

- **Severe Cracking** – You likely see commercials with potions, machines, and creams to try to get rid of severe foot cracking, peeling, and scaling, but the best way to remedy these issues is to seek professional care from a podiatrist. Sometimes this is caused by a severe infection and not what you may think.

Only a diagnosis can clear up any question so that you treat it correctly.

- **Blisters** – A blister can occur due to poor fitting socks and shoes. If you get blisters every time you try to walk or exercise for any period of time, see your podiatrist because they can help you know how to work with your feet to avoid this problem.

- **Possible Infection** – If your feet are swollen, red, tender or hot you may have an infection. See a doctor if you have pus, discharge, or other sores as those can be a sign of infection. Any problems that do not improve after a couple of weeks of home treatment should be treated by a doctor.

Any changes in your normal foot health will need to be diagnosed by a medical professional. If it's okay with your doctor you might want to try some spa treatments and/or reflexology.

Spa Treatments & Reflexology

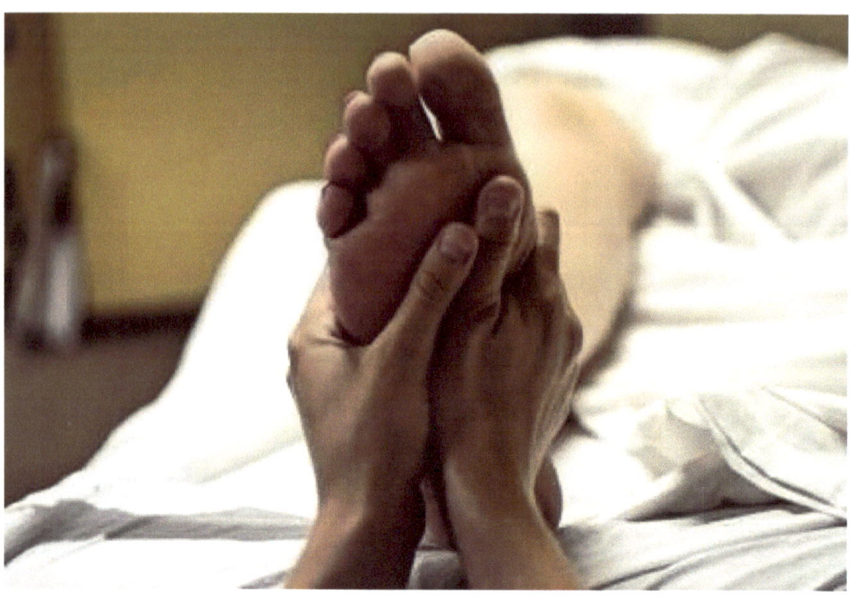

Find a local spa that offers foot spa treatments with reflexology. Reflexology is a system of massage on the feet, hands, and head. Reflexologists believe that reflex points in these parts of the body can be traced to every other part of the body.

A simple Google search can reveal reflexology charts which show what parts of your feet, hands, and head being massaged affects other parts of your body. Whether the theory lives up to its hype or not may be in question but there is no question that people get a lot of relief with spa treatments and reflexology.

Usually, if you go to a spa that practices reflexology for feet it'll work something like this:

Foot Soak

You'll first get a nice foot soak and probably a wash. Often your feet will be soaked in hot water or very warm water. If you have diabetes inform your practitioner because you want to avoid soaking your feet in too hot of water if this is the case.

Different spas do it differently but you'll likely soak your feet in something like tea or essential oils or a combination. It's thought that various essential oils can relax you and help treat painful conditions and even infection when done properly.

Usually, you'll soak your feet for about ten to twenty minutes. After that, they'll probably wash, or at least dry, your feet before they start the massage part.

Pressure Point Massage

The technician has been well trained in reflexology and knows how to massage your feet properly. You shouldn't experience a lot of pain. If you do, tell your reflexologist how you're feeling. Many people fall asleep while they're getting the pressure treatment.

Often, you'll let the reflexologist know about the health issues you're having outside of just your feet. For example, if you have sinus issues, the reflexologist knows right where to apply pressure on your feet to help soothe your sinus issues. The reflexologist may use hands, stones, sticks, and other tools to help get to your pressure points.

The other thing is that any type of massage, including reflexology, helps with blood flow to the feet. When you get good blood flow to your feet, your feet can heal easier. Blood brings oxygen and oxygen is needed to heal your feet.

Balance & Energy

The added benefit of reflexology is that your practitioner will also massage your legs. They'll do short and long massage strokes that helps bring circulation to the area, which will make your legs feel wonderful too. Some spas add in a sugar scrub. This is also good for helping with blood flow, which will help with any pain and swelling you're experiencing.

Most people experience increased energy and balance after getting spa treatments along with reflexology. The reason is that when your feet feel good your entire body feels good. When you feel good you're more likely to take care of yourself, eat right, and get plenty of exercises which will, in the end, improve your foot health.

If you can afford to get spa treatments and reflexology treatments try to do it at least monthly, but weekly might be better if you can swing it. What you save in health care costs can truly make it worth it.

Home Spa Treatments for Your Feet

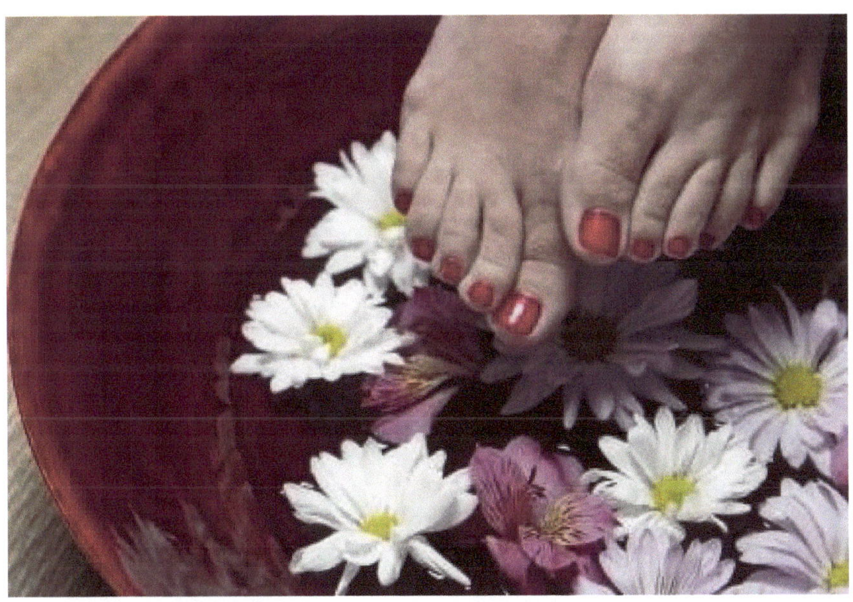

If you don't want to spend the money for a professional to help you with your feet, there are some home spa treatments you can do. If you can't do it yourself, you can have a girls' night party and help each other get it done. Spouses can also work together to help with each other's foot care. It'll bring you closer and everyone will feel great.

The Soak

You can soak your feet in a brathtub or you can buy one of the many foot spa soaking solutions available at Walmart, Target, as well as Amazon.

The feet are tender and need careful treatment. Try not to soak too often. Soaking your feet too often can backfire and make your skin drier.

Ensure that you do not use super-hot water as it's drying and bad for your circulation. It will dry your feet out more. You want the water to be comfortably warm. What you soak your feet in depends on your issues, your personal allergies, and preferences.

Soak for no more than 20 minutes once a week, unless a doctor has directed you to do otherwise.

Let's look at a few ideas.

Epsom Salt – Adding Epsom salt to your soaking water will help your tired, achy and swollen feet by helping your body let go of the excess water it's hanging onto. Use about ½ cup Epsom Salt to each gallon of water used to soak your feet.

Baking Soda – Put about ¼ cup baking soda to a gallon of water to soak your feet. This will work to help soothe dry, itchy skin, plus clean wounds if you have any. You can even make a paste of baking soda and water to create a scrub for your feet to get rid of hard callouses.

Peppermint Soak – If your feet feel hot, tired, and sore, and as long as you don't have any cuts or problems like that, you can create a peppermint soak that will energize your feet and soothe tired muscles. Add about 4 drops of peppermint essential oil to each gallon of soaking water.

Lavender Soak – This one is fun for the tub. Lavender is very relaxing because it has such a soothing aroma. People who can't handle peppermint will often enjoy lavender essential oils. Just one sniff and you will start to feel relaxed.

Vinegar Soak – This can help soothe dry cracked skin and disinfect imperfections too. Vinegar can help get rid of athlete's foot, foot odor, and toenail fungus. Just put about a ¼ cup into each gallon of soaking water. The best type of vinegar to use is regular apple cider vinegar.

Milk Soak – If you have super dry skin, a milk soak might be just what you need. Just add 1-part milk to 2-parts water for the milk soak. If you like you can add essential oils to the soak to add an extra component to your soak. Heating the milk first will ensure that the water stays warm too.

Don't soak more than weekly or you might cause your feet to become drier. Always dry your feet completely when you're done. You don't want left over moisture to be a breeding ground for bacteria and fungus.

If your feet are painful daily, even if you don't work on your feet all day, talk to a medical professional about ways to get relief without drying out your skin more. Treatments such as paraffin wax are known to be helpful for dry skin. However, if you have diabetes you should not do any of this without your doctor's approval.

The Massage

Give yourself a foot massage. You can get your spouse or a friend to do it for you, or you can use various machines to help. Some of the foot spa systems that you can buy have vibrating bottoms that help massage.

Foot Exercises to Do at Home

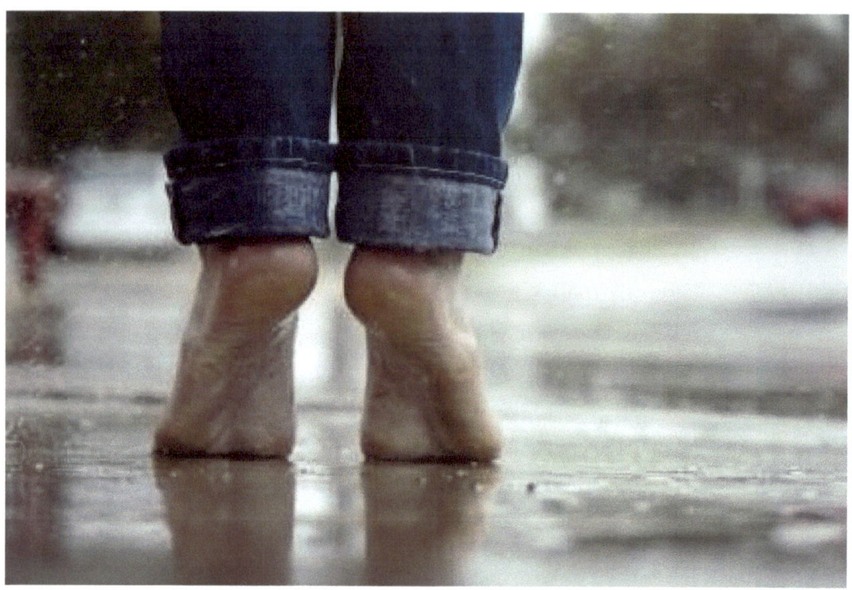

One way to keep your feet healthy is by exercising them. A good exercise, that most people can do, is walk. But, if you are having issues walking, due to painful feet, worn or poorly fitting shoes, you might want to try some of the following exercises to get some relief.

- **The Point** – From your ankle, flex your feet so that your foot is pointing down. Try to make a point with your big toe. Lift your foot up, then push back down into a point. You can do this sitting or standing. This helps stretch the muscles in the bottom of your feet. Stretching can help improve blood flow which can decrease pain.

- **Heel Lift** – If you're standing for long periods of time, this is a good exercise to do at that time. It will help relieve the pain and give you great muscle tone in your calves. Just lift your heels so that you're standing on the balls of your feet. Keep the form for about 5 to 10 seconds. Do these five to ten times in a row.

- **The Squeeze** – If you have hammer toe you'll need to do this exercise. Put something between your toes, such as the foam toe separators you use when you apply nail polish to them. Then squeeze your toes together. Do 10 five second reps for each foot.

- **Ball Roll** – Get a tennis ball, place it under the ball of your foot and roll it around for a few seconds, up to two minutes. The can help relieve pain if your arch hurts, you have foot cramps or even heel pain.

- **Arch Stretch** – Using a towel, position the towel so that you're holding it with both hands and your foot is cradled in the middle of the towel. Simultaneously, press your foot into the towel while also pulling the towel towards you to provide resistance. Do ten reps, holding 10 seconds each.

- **Wall Stretch** – This works the same as the Arch Stretch, but instead of using a towel, use the side of a wall. Go to a wall, lay down and put your heel on the floor with your toes pointed upwards. Press your toes into the wall which will stretch your arch too.

Doing any of these exercises will help you care for your feet better. When you have less foot pain, and fewer problems, due to the actions you take today, you'll know that you've done the right thing for your foot health.

Conclusion

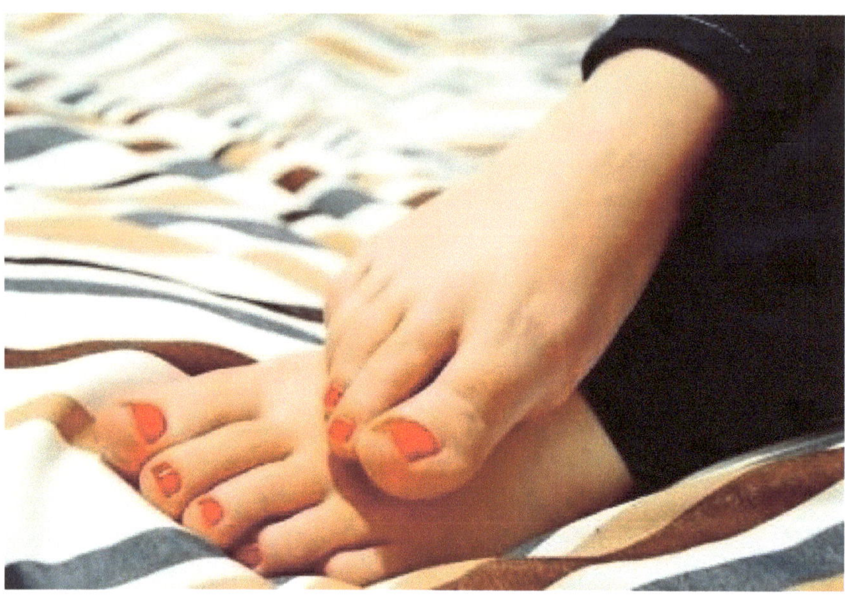

It's clear that taking care of your feet is important for overall good health care. Whether you seek professional assistance through podiatry, spa treatments, reflexology, or do it yourself, you can ensure that your feet carry you well through life if you pamper and take care of them.

If you do have health issues already, check with your doctor before trying anything at home. If you're otherwise healthy and don't have foot pain yet, then you should be fine to go with home health care or spa treatments with reflexology.

Just be sure to check that anyone who is working on your feet has the right credentials so they know how to do it right and don't cause more harm. This is especially true at spas.

Remember to speak up about what you want so you can truly get foot pampering that makes a difference.

About the Author

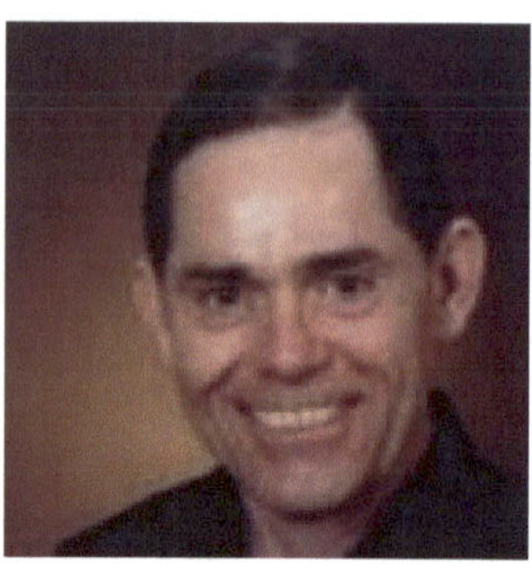

I have published over 125 books on Amazon for Kindle, CreateSpace and other publishing platforms.

While most of my books are on health and fitness in general, as I age (now 65) at the time of this writing) my topics of interest are geared toward aging baby boomers and older.

Besides my own writing, I also ghostwrite ebooks, books, reports, articles, blogs and do Kindle conversions for clients on a variety of topics.

Today my wife and I are retired from our careers and live in Gold Canyon, AZ. I now write as a retirement business where you'll find me happily sitting in my office typing away on my laptop as I work on my next book or ghostwriting project . . . that is if we are not traveling on a cruise ship - our new-found mode of travel.

For a complete list of my books published, go to my Amazon **Author Page** at: **https://www.amazon.com/Ron-Kness/e/B0072M6PYO**

www.ingramcontent.com/pod-product-compliance
Lightning Source LLC
Chambersburg PA
CBHW040248240726
48664CB00001B/308